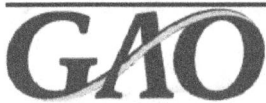

United States Government Accountability Office

Report to Congressional Committees

May 2013

MEDICARE IMAGING ACCREDITATION

Establishing Minimum National Standards and an Oversight Framework Would Help Ensure Quality and Safety of Advanced Diagnostic Imaging Services

GAO-13-246

GAO Highlights

Highlights of GAO-13-246, a report to congressional committees

May 2013

MEDICARE IMAGING ACCREDITATION

Establishing Minimum National Standards and an Oversight Framework Would Help Ensure Quality and Safety of Advanced Diagnostic Imaging Services

Why GAO Did This Study

MIPPA required that beginning January 1, 2012, suppliers that produce the images for ADI services, such as physician offices and independent diagnostic testing facilities, be accredited by an organization approved by CMS. MIPPA directed GAO to conduct a preliminary report on the accreditation requirement in 2013 and a final report in 2014.

In this report, GAO assessed (1) CMS's standards for accreditation of ADI suppliers, and (2) CMS's oversight of the accreditation requirement. To assess CMS's standards and oversight, GAO reviewed CMS regulations related to MIPPA, interviewed and reviewed information from CMS and CMS-approved accrediting organizations, and reviewed information on recommended standards for ADI accreditation from 11 organizations with imaging expertise.

What GAO Recommends

To help ensure that ADI suppliers provide safe and high-quality imaging to Medicare beneficiaries, GAO recommends that the Administrator of CMS determine the content of and publish minimum national standards for the accreditation of ADI suppliers; develop an oversight framework for evaluating accrediting organization performance; and develop more specific requirements for accrediting organization audits and clarify guidance on immediate-jeopardy deficiencies. The Department of Health and Human Services, which oversees CMS, concurred with GAO's recommendations.

View GAO-13-246. For more information, contact James Cosgrove at (202) 512-7114 or cosgrovej@gao.gov.

What GAO Found

The Centers for Medicare & Medicaid Services (CMS) did not establish minimum national standards for the accreditation of suppliers of advanced diagnostic imaging (ADI) services, which cover the production of images for computed tomography, magnetic resonance imaging, and nuclear medicine services. While CMS adopted the broad criteria from the Medicare Improvements for Patients and Providers Act of 2008 (MIPPA) for ADI accreditation, it relied on the three accrediting organizations it selected to establish their own standards for quality and safety. To establish a framework for assessing the ADI standards currently in use, GAO developed a list of nine standards based on recommendations from 11 organizations with imaging expertise from which GAO obtained information. Two of the three accrediting organizations that CMS selected use all nine standards, while the third organization uses six of the nine standards. For example, while two of the organizations evaluate suppliers' patient images, the third said that it instead assesses suppliers' compliance with other standards necessary to maintain image quality, such as those related to inspection and testing of imaging equipment. As a result of these significant differences among the accrediting organizations, which arise from the lack of minimum national standards, important aspects of imaging, such as qualifications of technologists and medical directors and the quality of clinical images, are difficult for CMS to monitor and assess. Nine of the 11 organizations with imaging expertise and representatives from all three accrediting organizations recommended that CMS adopt minimum national standards. CMS drafted standards in 2010, but did not publish them because the agency was focused on other priorities.

CMS's current oversight for the accreditation requirement is limited, as the agency focused its initial oversight efforts on ensuring that claims were paid only to accredited suppliers. Although CMS is responsible for evaluating the performance of accrediting organizations, the agency has not developed an oversight framework that would enable it to monitor and measure performance. CMS has not established specific performance expectations or developed plans for the validation audits of accredited suppliers as described in its regulations. Our previous work has shown that such independent evaluations are one of the most effective techniques CMS has to collect information about whether serious deficiencies are being identified. In addition, CMS's guidance to accrediting organizations on mid-cycle audits and serious care problems is limited. For example, CMS requires accrediting organizations to conduct mid-cycle audits to help ensure accredited suppliers maintain compliance for the 3-year accreditation cycle, but did not specify minimum expectations for this task, such as the minimum number or percentage of audits required or the types of supplier activities that should be assessed. In addition, two of the three accrediting organizations reported that CMS's guidance on identifying and reporting deficiencies that pose immediate jeopardy to Medicare beneficiaries or suppliers' staff was unclear. A CMS official stated that the accreditation requirement had been in operation for less than 1 year at the time of GAO's review, and reported that responsibility for oversight of the accreditation requirement was in the process of being transferred to another group within the agency.

United States Government Accountability Office

Contents

Letter		1
	Background	5
	CMS Currently Relies on Each Accrediting Organization to Establish Its Own Standards	10
	CMS's Current Oversight Is Limited	15
	Conclusions	20
	Recommendations for Executive Action	20
	Agency and Third Party Comments and Our Evaluation	21
Appendix I	Comments for the Department of Health and Human Services	25
Appendix II	GAO Contact and Staff Acknowledgments	27

Tables

	Table 1: Information about CMS-Designated Accrediting Organizations	8
	Table 2: Accrediting Organizations' Use of Advanced Diagnostic Imaging Standards Recommended by Organizations with Imaging Expertise	14

Abbreviations

ACR	American College of Radiology
ADI	advanced diagnostic imaging
CMS	Centers for Medicare & Medicaid Services
CT	computed tomography
FDA	Food and Drug Administration
HHS	Department of Health and Human Services
IAC	Intersocietal Accreditation Commission
MedPAC	Medicare Payment Advisory Commission
MIPPA	Medicare Improvements for Patients and Providers Act of 2008
MQSA	Mammography Quality Standards Act of 1992
MRI	magnetic resonance imaging
NM	nuclear medicine
NPI	national provider identifier
PECOS	Provider Enrollment, Chain and Ownership System
PET	positron emission tomography
TJC	The Joint Commission

This is a work of the U.S. government and is not subject to copyright protection in the United States. The published product may be reproduced and distributed in its entirety without further permission from GAO. However, because this work may contain copyrighted images or other material, permission from the copyright holder may be necessary if you wish to reproduce this material separately.

GAO
U.S. GOVERNMENT ACCOUNTABILITY OFFICE
441 G St. N.W.
Washington, DC 20548

May 31, 2013

Congressional Committees

Advanced diagnostic imaging (ADI) services, such as computed tomography (CT), magnetic resonance imaging (MRI), and nuclear medicine (NM), allow physicians to diagnose life-threatening diseases like cancer and heart disease with greater speed and precision.[1] However, quality problems such as inadequately trained technologists or poorly functioning equipment can lead to duplicative or inaccurate imaging tests, unnecessary exposure to radiation, missed or inaccurate diagnoses, and inappropriate treatment. To address concerns regarding the quality of imaging services provided to Medicare beneficiaries, the Medicare Payment Advisory Commission (MedPAC)[2] recommended that the Centers for Medicare & Medicaid Services (CMS), which administers the Medicare program, establish standards for imaging suppliers and select accrediting organizations to verify compliance with those standards. The Medicare Improvements for Patients and Providers Act of 2008 (MIPPA) required that beginning January 1, 2012, suppliers of the technical component of ADI services be accredited by a designated accrediting organization in order to receive Medicare payment for these services.[3] This requirement applies to ADI suppliers paid under the physician fee schedule, such as physician offices and independent diagnostic testing facilities.[4] MIPPA outlined broad criteria that accrediting organizations should use to evaluate ADI suppliers, such as standards for qualifications of personnel and standards to ensure the safety of beneficiaries and staff.

---

[1]There are six types of medical imaging capabilities, referred to as modalities: CT, MRI, NM, ultrasound, X-ray and other standard imaging, and procedures that use imaging, such as using ultrasound to localize a needle when performing a biopsy.

[2]MedPAC is an independent federal body that advises Congress on issues affecting the Medicare program. See MedPAC, *Report to the Congress: Medicare Payment Policy* (Washington, D.C.: March 2005).

[3]Pub. L. No. 110-275, § 135(a), 122 Stat. 2494, 2532 (codified at 42 U.S.C.§ 1395m(e)). Medicare divides payment for ADI services into two components: the technical component, which is the production of the image, and the professional component, which is a physician's interpretation of the image and report on the findings.

[4]MIPPA accreditation does not apply to the technical component of ADI services provided in Medicare settings not paid under the physician fee schedule, such as hospital inpatient or outpatient departments.

CMS administers the MIPPA accreditation requirement on behalf of the Secretary of Health and Human Services and has selected three organizations to serve as designated accrediting organizations—the American College of Radiology (ACR), the Intersocietal Accreditation Commission (IAC), and The Joint Commission (TJC). CMS is also responsible for overseeing accreditation organizations' compliance with MIPPA regulations.[5] CMS officials indicated that the overall goal of the program is to improve the quality of ADI services.

MIPPA directed us to report on the effect of the accreditation requirement administered by CMS. We are required to issue a preliminary report in 2013 and a final report in 2014. In this preliminary report, we assessed (1) CMS's standards for accreditation of ADI suppliers, and (2) CMS's oversight of the accreditation requirement.[6]

To assess CMS's standards for accreditation of ADI suppliers, we reviewed federal regulations related to the MIPPA accreditation requirement, reviewed applications from accreditation organizations, and interviewed CMS officials. In addition, we interviewed representatives from each of the three accrediting organizations[7] and collected information on the standards and processes they used to assess ADI suppliers' compliance with those standards. To establish a framework for assessing the standards currently in use, we also obtained information on recommended standards for ADI suppliers from 11 organizations with imaging expertise. These included either organizations that represent individuals that order, perform, or interpret images such as national medical specialty societies or other organizations that focus on the quality

---

[5]Federal agencies in addition to CMS have regulatory responsibility for imaging devices and services, including FDA and the Nuclear Regulatory Commission. FDA is responsible for establishing quality standards for mammography equipment and ensuring that manufacturers of radiation-emitting imaging equipment are in compliance with applicable performance standards. The Nuclear Regulatory Commission oversees the medical uses of nuclear materials used by physicians, hospitals, and others through licensing, inspection, and enforcement programs.

[6]In the final report, we plan to examine the effect of the accreditation requirement on ADI services on the basis of data available in 2013. This could include the effect of accreditation on utilization, quality, and beneficiary access to ADI services.

[7]At the time of our review, CMS was in the process of reviewing an application for another accrediting organization.

or safety of ADI services.[8] We identified these 11 organizations through a review of relevant industry and scholarly articles, government reports, and congressional hearings. To identify recommended standards, we used a structured questionnaire to ask these 11 organizations about the specific types of standards they would expect for the accreditation of ADI suppliers. On the basis of our review of their responses, we derived a list of specific standards or practices supported by at least 5 of the 11 organizations—which we refer to as recommended standards—that could be used by accrediting organizations to evaluate ADI suppliers.[9] We then determined whether each of the three CMS-designated accrediting organizations used the recommended standards in its accreditation process. Because we used a sample of organizations with imaging expertise, the standards they identified do not represent the full range of possible standards for the accreditation of ADI suppliers, but rather provide a framework for comparing the standards used by the accrediting organizations selected by CMS.

To assess the effectiveness of CMS's oversight of the accreditation requirement, we analyzed the laws and regulations that define CMS's role and authority. On the basis of our review of CMS's oversight authority and the agency's goal for accreditation to improve the quality of ADI services, we reviewed three components of CMS oversight: (1) mechanisms for ensuring payment is made only to accredited suppliers; (2) processes for evaluating accrediting organizations' performance; and (3) policies for ensuring that ADI suppliers maintain compliance with standards for the duration of the accreditation cycle and that serious care problems are identified and corrected. To supplement our review of CMS oversight, we also collected information on accreditation results from each of the three

---

[8] We obtained information from the following organizations: The American Academy of Neurology, the American Academy of Orthopaedic Surgeons, the American Board of Orthopaedic Surgery, the American Association of Physicists in Medicine, the American College of Cardiology, the American Society of Nuclear Cardiology, the American Society of Radiologic Technologists, the Conference on Radiation Control Program Directors, the Medical Imaging & Technology Alliance, the Radiology Outcomes Research Laboratory at the University of California, San Francisco, and the Society for Nuclear Medicine and Molecular Imaging.

[9] The 11 organizations have expertise in different areas of ADI services; as a result, not all organizations commented on all sections of the questionnaire or on all three modalities. For example, the American Board of Orthopaedic Surgery recommended standards related to the qualifications of medical directors or supervising physicians, but not procedures to ensure that equipment meets performance specifications.

accrediting organizations, including the percentage of suppliers that were not granted accreditation after the first attempt, as well as the types of deficiencies most frequently identified.

To provide context for our findings, we also compared CMS's standards and oversight mechanisms for the ADI accreditation requirement to those used by the Food and Drug Administration (FDA) to ensure the quality of another type of imaging—mammography.[10] We previously reported that FDA's implementation of the Mammography Quality Standards Act of 1992 (MQSA) had a positive effect on the quality of mammography without negatively affecting access to these services.[11] In addition to reviewing our prior work on mammography, we reviewed the laws and regulations that define FDA's responsibilities for oversight of mammography and its standards for selected accrediting bodies.

We conducted this performance audit from May 2012 to May 2013 in accordance with generally accepted government auditing standards. Those standards require that we plan and perform the audit to obtain sufficient, appropriate evidence to provide a reasonable basis for our findings and conclusions based on our audit objectives. We believe that the evidence obtained provides a reasonable basis for our findings and conclusions based on our audit objectives.

---

[10]In response to concerns about the safety, accuracy, and quality of mammography—an imaging service that uses X-rays to detect small tumors and breast abnormalities—the Mammography Quality Standards Act of 1992 (MQSA) and the Mammography Quality Standards Reauthorization Acts of 1998 and 2004 were enacted. Pub. L. No. 102-539, 106 Stat. 3547; Pub. L. No. 105-248, 112 Stat. 1864; Pub. L. No. 108-365, 118 Stat. 1738 (pertinent provisions of all three laws codified at 42 U.S.C. § 263b). FDA administers the requirements of MQSA on behalf of the Department of Health and Human Services (HHS).

[11]See GAO, *Mammography Services: Impact of Federal Legislation on Quality, Access, and Health Outcomes,* GAO/HEHS-98-11 (Washington, D.C.: Oct. 21, 1997).

Background

Imaging Modalities

MIPPA defines ADI services to include diagnostic CT, MRI, and NM, including positron emission tomography (PET).[12] CT is an imaging modality that uses ionizing radiation and computers to produce cross-sectional images of internal organs and body structures. MRI is an imaging modality that uses powerful magnets, radio waves, and computers to create cross-sectional images of internal body tissues. NM is the use of radioactive materials in conjunction with an imaging modality to produce images that show both structure and function within the body. During an NM service, such as a PET scan, a patient is administered a small amount of radioactive substance, called a radiopharmaceutical or radiotracer, which is subsequently tracked by a radiation detector outside the body to render time-lapse images of the radioactive material as it moves through the body.

Imaging equipment that uses ionizing radiation—such as CT and NM—poses greater potential short- and long-term health risks to patients than other imaging modalities, such as ultrasound. This is because ionizing radiation has enough energy to potentially damage DNA and thus increase a person's lifetime risk of developing cancer. In addition, exposure to very high doses of this radiation can cause short-term injuries, such as burns or hair loss. Each of the modalities using ionizing radiation uses different amounts of such radiation. For example, conventional X-ray imaging, in which X-rays are projected through a patient's body to produce two-dimensional pictures of organs and tissue, uses relatively low amounts of radiation in order to render a diagnostic-quality radiographic image. Because CT and NM services can involve repeated or extended exposure to ionizing radiation, they are associated with the administration of higher radiation doses than conventional X-ray imaging systems. In its 2010 initiative to reduce unnecessary radiation, FDA reported that the effective dose from a CT is roughly equivalent to 100 to 800 chest X-rays, whereas a NM service is equivalent to 10 to

---

[12]MIPPA also provided for the inclusion of certain other diagnostic imaging services as specified by CMS in consultation with physician specialty organizations and other stakeholders.

2,050 chest X-rays.[13] Because using a higher radiation dose can produce higher-resolution images, FDA advises that an optimal radiation dose is one that is as low as reasonably achievable while maintaining sufficient image quality to meet the clinical need. Although MRIs do not use ionizing radiation, they pose other potential dangers; for example, magnetic fields from the MRI unit can result in a "projectile effect," in which magnetic material, such as the metal in oxygen cylinders or wheelchairs, can be pulled suddenly and—often violently—toward the imaging equipment at times while a patient lies in the center of the magnet and while medical personnel are attending to the patient.

MIPPA Requirements

MIPPA requires the establishment of procedures to ensure that accrediting organizations include standards specific to each imaging modality for ADI suppliers in the following five areas: (1) qualifications of medical personnel who are not physicians and who furnish the technical component of ADI services; (2) qualifications and responsibilities of medical directors and supervising physicians; (3) procedures to ensure that equipment used in furnishing the technical component of ADI services meets performance specifications; (4) procedures to ensure the safety of beneficiaries and staff; and (5) establishment and maintenance of a quality-assurance and quality-control program that ensures the reliability, clarity, and accuracy of the technical quality of diagnostic images produced by suppliers.[14]

---

[13]The radiation doses vary based on the type of imaging exam conducted. For example, a CT scan of the head uses less radiation than a CT scan of the abdomen. See FDA, *Initiative to Reduce Unnecessary Radiation Exposure from Medical Imaging* (Silver Spring, Md.: February 2010), accessed January 6, 2013, http://www.fda.gov/Radiation-EmittingProducts/RadiationSafety/RadiationDoseReduction/ucm199994.htm.

[14]MIPPA also provided for the inclusion of any additional standards CMS determines appropriate. Throughout this report, we use the term technologists to refer to nonphysician medical personnel who furnish the technical component of ADI services. We use the term medical directors to refer to medical directors and supervising physicians because, under applicable federal regulations, these may be the same person. 42 C.F.R. § 414.68 (c)(1)(ii) (2012).

MIPPA accreditation applies only to suppliers paid under the Medicare physician fee schedule that provide the technical component of ADI services.[15] Suppliers paid under the physician fee schedule include physician offices and independent diagnostic testing facilities, which are independent of a hospital or physician office and provide only diagnostic outpatient services. MIPPA accreditation does not apply to the technical component of ADI services provided in Medicare settings not paid under the physician fee schedule, such as hospital inpatient or outpatient departments.[16] To become accredited, ADI suppliers must first select one of the three CMS-designated organizations and pay the organization an accreditation fee. Among other things, CMS requires accrediting organizations to evaluate ADI suppliers during the initial application regarding compliance with MIPPA requirements—such as qualifications of personnel—as well as during mid-cycle audit procedures to ensure suppliers maintain compliance for the duration of the accreditation cycle, which is a 3-year period. ACR and IAC primarily grant initial accreditation through an online application and review of suppliers' documents, while TJC uses an online application but also conducts an on-site visit for each supplier prior to granting accreditation.

Information about the three accrediting organizations that CMS has designated for ADI suppliers—ACR, IAC, and TJC—follows in table 1.

---

[15]The technical component of the Medicare payment is designed to cover the cost of performing an imaging test, including the costs for equipment, supplies, and nonphysician staff, whereas the professional component is designed to cover the provider's time in interpreting the image and writing a report on the findings. The technical and professional components of imaging can be billed separately if the performing and interpreting providers are different, and can be billed together on what is called a global claim if the same provider performs and interprets the imaging service.

[16]Hospitals must comply with Medicare's "conditions of participation" rules, which include general standards for imaging equipment and facilities, staff qualifications, patient safety, record keeping, and proper handling of radioactive materials.

Table 1: Information about CMS-Designated Accrediting Organizations

	American College of Radiology (ACR)	Intersocietal Accreditation Commission (IAC)	The Joint Commission (TJC)
Suppliers accredited, by modality[a]			
CT suppliers	3,636	1,361	64
MRI suppliers	4,035	1,052	68
NM suppliers	2,488	6,554	23
PET suppliers	1,009	635	7
Total unique suppliers	**6,855**	**8,491**	**98**
Accreditation fee (dollars)	1,800 to 2,400 (per unit of imaging equipment; varies by modality)[b]	2,600 to 3,800 (per application; varies by modality)[c]	8,740 to 14,890 (per facility; varies by patient volume and includes an on-site visit for all applicants)[d]

Source: GAO analysis of information from CMS and CMS-designated accrediting organizations.

[a]The number of accredited suppliers was provided by CMS on January 3, 2013. Each supplier may have multiple locations. The sum of the number of accredited suppliers by modality does not equal the total number of unique suppliers because some suppliers provide more than one imaging modality.

[b]Discounted fees are available for facilities with more than one imaging unit and multiple modalities. Additional fees of $780 to $3,315 apply for a phantom, a solid object designed to mimic critical imaging characteristics of patients, such as bone and tissue, that is imaged using suppliers' equipment to help assess performance parameters such as resolution and image uniformity. The price varies depending on the specific phantom and modality.

[c]Application fee varies by modality and covers the first unit of imaging equipment for MRI and CT; the fee for NM and PET covers all of the equipment. For MRI and CT, discounted fees are available for each additional unit for facilities with more than one imaging unit. For all modalities, there is a discount for facilities with more than one site.

[d]Additional fees apply for suppliers with more than one location or that require additional specialists. TJC accreditation for ADI is part of the accreditation program for ambulatory care facilities; its costs are based on the number of patient visits rather than on each imaging unit or modality. TJC accreditation fees include an on-site visit fee for all applicants and an annual fee billed each year during the 3-year accreditation cycle.

CMS Oversight

CMS has several responsibilities to ensure the quality of ADI services paid under Medicare's physician fee schedule. In addition to selecting accrediting organizations, CMS is responsible for ensuring that Medicare payment is made only to ADI suppliers accredited by a CMS-approved accrediting organization. MIPPA requires CMS to oversee the accrediting organizations and authorizes CMS to modify the list of selected accrediting organizations, if necessary. Federal regulations specify that CMS may conduct "validation audits" of accredited ADI suppliers and provide for the withdrawal of CMS approval of an accrediting organization at any time if CMS determines that the accrediting organization no longer adequately ensures that ADI suppliers meet or exceed Medicare requirements.[17] In addition, accrediting organizations are required to report serious care problems that pose immediate jeopardy to a beneficiary or to the general public to CMS within 2 business days of identifying such problems.[18] CMS also has ongoing requirements for accrediting organizations; among other things, accrediting organizations are responsible for using mid-cycle audit procedures, such as unannounced site visits, to ensure that accredited suppliers maintain compliance with MIPPA's requirements for the duration of the accreditation cycle.

FDA Oversight of Mammography	MQSA, as amended by the Mammography Quality Standards Reauthorization Acts of 1998 and 2004, established national quality standards for mammography to help ensure the high quality of images and image interpretation that mammography facilities produce. Under MQSA, FDA—acting on behalf of the Department of Health and Human Services (HHS)—has several responsibilities to ensure the quality of mammography:

- establishing quality standards for mammography equipment, personnel, and practices;

- ensuring that all mammography facilities are accredited by an FDA-approved accrediting body and have obtained a certificate permitting them to provide mammography services from FDA or an FDA-approved certification agency;[19]

- ensuring that all mammography equipment is evaluated at least annually by a qualified medical physicist and that all mammography facilities receive an annual compliance inspection from an FDA-approved inspector; and

- performing annual evaluations of the accreditation bodies and certification agencies.

---

[17] 42 C.F.R. § 414.68(g), (h) (2012).

[18] 42 C.F.R. § 414.68(g), (2012).

[19] Mammography facilities operated by the Department of Veterans Affairs are excluded from FDA review.

CMS Currently Relies on Each Accrediting Organization to Establish Its Own Standards

CMS did not establish minimum national standards for ADI accreditation, and instead required each accrediting organization to establish its own specific standards for quality and safety of ADI services. In 2009, CMS solicited applications from accrediting organizations and outlined the information that needed to be furnished by each organization to be considered for approval. As part of its application requirements, CMS adopted the broad MIPPA criteria for ADI accreditation and required each accrediting organization to provide a detailed description of how its standards satisfy these requirements.[20] For example, CMS required each accrediting organization to have standards regarding qualifications for suppliers' technologists and medical directors, but allowed the accrediting organizations to establish their own minimum certification, experience, and continuing education requirements. In addition, CMS required accrediting organizations to provide documentation of other requirements, such as detailed information about the individuals who perform evaluations for accrediting organizations and a description of the organization's data management and analysis capabilities in support of its surveys and accreditation decisions. CMS received three applications from its solicitation and in January 2010, the agency reported that an internal professional panel had reviewed the applications and determined that all three organizations provided sufficient evidence of their ability to accredit ADI suppliers on the basis of CMS's requirements.

CMS drafted more specific standards for the accreditation of ADI suppliers in 2010, but did not publish these standards or propose adopting them. A CMS official told us that the agency developed the draft standards in conjunction with FDA[21] and incorporated comments from each of the accrediting organizations. This official also told us that the draft standards were not put through the rulemaking process because the agency was focused on developing regulations for the Patient Protection and Affordable Care Act, which was enacted 2010. As of January 2013, these CMS standards remained in draft form, and officials told us that the agency did not have a specific timeline for publishing the standards in a

---

[20]Medicare Program: Payment Policies Under the Physician Fee Schedule and Other Revisions to Part B for CY 2010. 74 Fed. Reg. 61,738 (Nov. 25, 2009) (codified at 42 C.F.R. § 414.68(c)(1)(2012)).

[21]FDA collaborated with CMS to incorporate key quality-assurance practices into accreditation and participation criteria for imaging facilities as part of its ongoing efforts to reduce radiation exposure from imaging services. See FDA, *Initiative to Reduce Unnecessary Radiation Exposure from Medical Imaging.*

proposed rule. Representatives from the three approved accrediting organizations—as well as 9 of the 11 organizations with imaging expertise from which we obtained information—recommended that CMS adopt minimum national standards, which would help to ensure that all accredited ADI suppliers meet a minimum level of quality and safety. In addition, we have reported that the quality of mammography services improved under MQSA primarily as a result of setting national quality-assurance standards—such as those related to personnel qualifications and clinical image quality—and establishing enforcement mechanisms to ensure that the standards are met by all mammography providers.[22]

CMS's lack of similar minimum national standards may prevent it from ensuring that all accredited ADI suppliers meet a minimum level of quality and safety. We found that two of the three accrediting organizations used all nine recommended standards we assessed, while the third organization used six of the nine standards (see table 2).[23] For example, ACR and IAC standards require technologists and medical directors to meet minimum qualifications based on specific certification, experience, or continuing-education requirements, as recommended by organizations with expertise in imaging.[24] In contrast, TJC standards do not require technologists and medical directors to meet specified minimum qualifications, but rather require these personnel to meet applicable laws as well as to meet qualifications defined by the supplier to perform assigned responsibilities. However, TJC's guide for evaluating ADI services indicates that not all states require technologists to be certified and have ongoing education. Further, 1 of the 11 organizations with imaging expertise—the Radiology Outcomes Research Laboratory at the University of California, San Francisco—reported that there is wide

---

[22]See GAO/HEHS-98-11 and *Mammography Services: Initial Impact of New Federal Law Has Been Positive*, GAO/HEHS-96-17 (Washington, D.C.: Oct. 27, 1995).

[23]The list of recommended standards was derived from recommendations obtained from at least 5 of 11 organizations with imaging expertise about the specific types of standards that they would expect accrediting organizations to use.

[24]Nine of the 11 organizations with imaging expertise recommended specific minimum qualifications for technologists or medical directors, and 5 of the 11 organizations recommended minimum qualifications for both. As an example of such qualifications, ACR requires medical directors for MRI services to have certain specified qualifications, such as board certification from the American Board of Radiology and specified experience requirements, such as reading 300 exams over a 36-month period; in addition, medical directors must earn at least 15 hours of continuing medical education requirements over a 36-month period.

variation in state requirements for training and certification of technologists, and lack of training is widely recognized as a cause of significant errors in the provision of ADI services. Another of the 11 organizations, the American Society of Radiologic Technologists, reported that imaging services performed by individuals who are not experienced, educated, or certified in a specific imaging modality could compromise the quality of images or jeopardize the health or safety of supplier staff or Medicare beneficiaries.

In addition, prior to granting accreditation, both ACR and IAC evaluate suppliers' patient images (called "clinical images") to ensure that images meet specific criteria, as recommended by 8 of the 11 organizations with imaging expertise. One of the 8, the American College of Cardiology, called the review of clinical images an essential component for assessing the capability of imaging equipment and the proficiency of staff in acquiring images. ACR and IAC also evaluate suppliers' phantom images prior to granting accreditation, which are images of a solid object designed to mimic critical imaging characteristics of patients that are used for the assessment of certain performance parameters of imaging equipment, as recommended by 5 of the 11 organizations. One of the 5, the American Association of Physicists in Medicine, reported that phantom images permit more objective evaluations of ADI equipment performance and a standardized format against which the imaging performance of various facilities can be evaluated. Further, FDA-approved accrediting bodies are also required to review mammography suppliers' clinical and phantom images, and we have reported with regard to mammography that evaluating phantom images is one of the most important processes for testing equipment.[25]

TJC does not systematically evaluate suppliers' clinical or phantom images to ensure that images meet specific criteria, although TJC representatives reported assessing compliance with standards that require suppliers to identify and implement activities necessary to maintain the reliability, clarity, and accuracy of the technical quality of

---

[25]See GAO, *FDA's Mammography Inspections: While Some Problems Need Attention, Facility Compliance is Growing*, GAO/HEHS-97-25 (Washington, D.C.: Jan. 27, 1997). FDA also requires each accrediting body to annually conduct random clinical image reviews of at least 3 percent of the facilities the body accredits.

images.[26] According to TJC representatives, health care services are provided in an environment that must be comprehensively assessed, and no single checklist can fulfill this. For example, they reported that evaluating an image does not reveal anything about the systems that support imaging safety such as the adequacy of safety checks, equipment maintenance, expertise of staff, and whether there is a primacy on patient and staff safety that permeates the facility's culture and process. However, ADI suppliers have been delayed accreditation by ACR and IAC on the basis of problems with the quality of their clinical images, such as inadequate anatomic coverage or excessive artifacts.[27] We and others have reported that quality problems with medical images can have serious consequences, such as missed or inaccurate diagnoses or inappropriate treatment.[28] Despite the potential health consequences that can result from poor-quality images, there are currently no image review requirements or other national standards for ADI accreditation.

---

[26] Such standards include, for example, requiring suppliers to inspect, test, and maintain imaging equipment. In addition, TJC representatives told us that a radiologist on the team may review supplier clinical images, but a systematic evaluation of clinical images is not part of the organization's accreditation standards.

[27] Artifacts refer to any feature that appears in an image that is not present in the original imaged object. Artifacts may be caused by a variety of factors, such as improper operation by the technologist or patient movement. Image artifacts can obscure, and be mistaken for, pathology.

[28] See GAO/HEHS-98-11; MedPAC: *Report to the Congress: Medicare Payment Policy*; and *Examining the Appropriateness of Standards for Medical Imaging and Radiation Therapy Technologists: Testimony in Support of the Consistency, Accuracy, Responsibility and Excellence in Medical Imaging and Radiation Therapy Bill (H.R. 2104), Before the House Energy and Commerce Committee, Subcommittee on Health*, 112th Cong. (2012) (statement of Sal Martino, Chief Executive Officer, American Society of Radiologic Technologists).

Table 2: Accrediting Organizations' Use of Advanced Diagnostic Imaging Standards Recommended by Organizations with Imaging Expertise

Recommended standards[a]	American College of Radiology (ACR)	Intersocietal Accreditation Commission (IAC)	The Joint Commission (TJC)
Personnel qualifications			
Ensures that supplier technologists and medical directors meet minimum qualifications based on specified certification, experience or continuing education requirements[b]	✓	✓	[c]
Equipment performance			
Ensures that supplier conducts equipment maintenance and quality control tests as specified by the manufacturer	✓	✓	✓
Ensures that supplier medical physicist (or similarly qualified expert) evaluates equipment performance at least annually	✓	✓	✓
Evaluates supplier phantom images[d]	✓	✓	
Quality assurance			
Ensures that supplier has established a quality assurance program that evaluates specific components of performance such as image quality and peer review of image interpretation	✓	✓	✓
Evaluates supplier patient (clinical) images	✓	✓	
Ensures that supplier reviews whether patient images are clinically appropriate	✓	✓	✓
Safety			
Ensures that supplier maintains policies and procedures for patient and personnel safety as appropriate for the modality	✓	✓	✓
Ensures that supplier keeps radiation exposure as low as reasonably achievable for a quality image	✓	✓	✓

Source: GAO analysis of information from accrediting organizations and organizations with imaging expertise.

[a] The list of recommended standards above was derived from recommendations obtained from at least 5 of 11 organizations with imaging expertise about the specific types of standards that they would expect accrediting organizations to use.

[b] We use the term medical directors to refer to medical directors and supervising physicians because these may be the same person.

[c] TJC standards require technologists and medical directors to meet applicable laws as well as to meet qualifications defined by the supplier to perform assigned responsbilities. Its standards also require that licensed independent practitioners, such as radiologists and nonradiologist physicians, be licensed by the state or the Nuclear Regulatory Commission; however, documentation does not indicate whether these requirements apply specifically to technologists or medical directors and may not apply to all modalities.

[d] A phantom is a solid object designed to mimic critical imaging characteristics of patients, such as bone and tissue, that is imaged using suppliers' equipment to help assess performance parameters such as resolution and image uniformity.

A CMS official told us that each accrediting organization has unique strengths, and representatives from the three accrediting organizations cited examples of their organization's strengths. For example, an ACR representative told us that ACR systematically evaluates phantom images,[29] whereas IAC representatives told us that IAC evaluates suppliers' interpretive reports of images and the associated clinical findings. Representatives from TJC indicated that TJC's approach is holistic, using a tracer methodology to follow the care, treatment, or services received by patients.[30] According to TJC representatives, a checklist approach can be problematic because the processes used by suppliers to achieve their goals may differ, and innovations with respect to quality may occur faster than standards can be developed. In addition, TJC representatives pointed out that TJC is the only organization that conducts an on-site visit of each ADI supplier prior to accreditation, providing onsite education and offering suggestions for approaches and strategies that may help the supplier better meet the intent of the standards and, more importantly, improve performance.

CMS's Current Oversight Is Limited

CMS's oversight efforts have focused primarily on ensuring that only accredited suppliers' claims are paid; the agency does not have a systematic oversight process for other aspects of the ADI accreditation requirement. CMS has not developed a framework for evaluating accrediting organization performance, and its current guidance is insufficient to ensure that suppliers maintain compliance with standards for the duration of the accreditation cycle and to ensure that serious care problems are consistently identified and reported.

---

[29]ACR representatives told us that its physicists evaluate and score phantom images on the basis of performance criteria that the organization has specified for each modality. In contrast, representatives from IAC told us that its organization evaluates phantom images on the basis of criteria established by each supplier's quality improvement committee or the equipment manufacturer, or both.

[30]The tracer methodology is used during TJC's on-site survey to identify performance issues in one or more steps of the health care delivery process. TJC uses three types of tracers: (1) program-specific tracers, which identify safety concerns within different levels and types of care, treatment, or services; (2) individual tracers, which "trace" the care, treatment, or services received by individual patients; and (3) system tracers, which explore one specific system or process across the organization.

CMS's Oversight Efforts Have Focused on Ensuring That Only Accredited Suppliers Are Paid

CMS's oversight efforts have primarily focused on ensuring that only accredited suppliers' claims are paid. To ensure payment is made only to accredited suppliers, CMS officials told us that they require accrediting organizations to submit updated information about accredited suppliers on a weekly basis, including their national provider identifier (NPI), enrollment number, address, name, and dates of accreditation for each modality. They explained that these data are uploaded into the Medicare Provider Enrollment, Chain and Ownership System (PECOS)—CMS's centralized database for Medicare provider enrollment information—and are matched against all claims submitted by ADI suppliers. If the NPI on a supplier's claim does not match an accredited supplier listed in PECOS, the claim is denied. CMS officials told us that there were problems with accredited suppliers' claims being denied when the accreditation requirement first went into effect because suppliers used an incorrect NPI; however, CMS officials and representatives from two of the accrediting organizations reported that these issues generally have been resolved.

CMS Has Not Developed an Oversight Framework for Evaluating Accrediting Organization Performance

Although CMS is responsible for evaluating the performance of accrediting organizations, and CMS officials have indicated that its goal is to improve the quality of ADI services, it has not developed an oversight framework that would enable it to monitor and measure performance. A CMS official knowledgeable about the accreditation requirement stated that the requirement had been in effect for less than 1 year at the time of our review, and acknowledged that the agency's oversight process was not as robust as it could be. This official reported that primary responsibility for oversight of the accreditation requirement was in the process of being transferred from CMS's Center for Program Integrity to the Center for Clinical Standards and Quality.[31] Although the accreditation requirement became effective January 1, 2012, it has been enacted into law since 2008 and CMS had selected accrediting organizations in January 2010, providing the agency with nearly 2 years to develop a plan for evaluating their performance before the effective date of the requirement.

---

[31] In its comments on our draft report, the Department of Health and Human Services indicated that the transition to the Center for Clinical Standards and Quality would become effective April 1, 2013.

We found that as of January 2013, CMS had not yet established specific performance expectations or developed plans for conducting validation audits of accredited suppliers, which are one of the most effective techniques CMS has for collecting information about accrediting organization performance.[32] Federal regulations provide for audits of a representative sample of accredited suppliers, which enable CMS to validate the processes used by approved accrediting organizations. These regulations also note that CMS may notify an accrediting organization of its intent to withdraw approval for an accrediting organization on the basis of the disparity between its findings and those of the respective accrediting organization. Further, in the absence of minimum national standards, it is unclear what measures CMS would use in its audits to validate the accreditation process and determine whether services provided by accredited ADI suppliers meet a sufficient level of quality and safety.

In addition, CMS does not systematically collect or analyze readily available data to monitor accrediting organization performance. Collecting and analyzing information from accrediting organizations on accreditation results, such as the proportion of suppliers delayed accreditation and the types of care problems identified, could provide useful information about accrediting organization performance and help CMS ensure that accreditation is improving the quality and safety of ADI services. CMS does not systematically collect or analyze data on the proportion of suppliers that were not granted accreditation after the first attempt, and we found significant variation among accrediting organizations on the rates of these "delayed" accreditations. For calendar year 2012, IAC and ACR representatives reported that the proportion of CT suppliers delayed accreditation was 81 percent with IAC and 25 percent with ACR; likewise, the proportion of NM suppliers delayed accreditation was 60 percent with

---

[32]We have previously reported that a similar type of independent survey used by CMS is the most effective technique the agency has for assessing the ability of state agencies to identify serious deficiencies in nursing homes. See GAO, *Nursing Homes, Prevalence of Serious Quality Problems Remains Unacceptably High, Despite Some Decline.* GAO-03-1016T (Washington, D.C.: July 17, 2003) and *Nursing Home Care, Enhanced HCFA Oversight of State Programs Would Better Ensure Quality*, GAO/HEHS-00-6 (Washington, D.C.: Nov. 4, 1999).

IAC and 4 percent with ACR.[33] It is unclear whether these differences were due to actual variations in the quality of services provided by suppliers or to differences in approaches used by accrediting organizations to enforce compliance with their standards. Similarly, CMS does not define the care problems, or "deficiencies," that may be identified by accrediting organizations that can result in delayed or denied accreditations, nor does it systematically collect information about or analyze the deficiencies identified. We found wide variation in the types of deficiencies most frequently identified by each accrediting organization during the accreditation process, which raises questions about whether organizations are consistently identifying care problems. For example, ACR most frequently identified problems with suppliers failing to submit required information, including clinical images of diagnostic quality; IAC most frequently identified problems with the interpretive reports written by physicians; and TJC most frequently identified problems on a wider range of issues, including problems with clinical privileges, equipment maintenance, medication management, infection control, and leadership.

CMS Guidance on Mid-Cycle Audits and Identification of Serious Care Problems Is Limited

Although CMS requires accrediting organizations to conduct mid-cycle audits of accredited suppliers—including unannounced site visits—to help ensure they maintain compliance for the duration of the accreditation cycle, CMS does not specify minimum expectations for this task, such as the minimum number or percentage of audits required or the types of supplier activities that should be assessed during such audits. We found that the mid-cycle audits conducted by accrediting organizations varied in number and type. ACR conducted unannounced site visits for approximately 1 percent of its accredited suppliers in 2012, but ACR intends to increase this amount to approximately 15 percent in 2013. IAC representatives stated that they ensure that all accredited suppliers undergo at least one unannounced site visit or a performance audit—which requires accredited suppliers to submit specified documentation including clinical images, interpretive reports, and quality-improvement documentation—to ensure continued compliance with IAC standards over

---

[33]We did not include TJC because of its small number of suppliers accredited. However, TJC representatives reported that they also delay accreditation when deficiencies are identified and do not grant accreditation until suppliers are in compliance with their standards.

the 3-year accreditation period.[34] TJC representatives stated that they conduct unannounced site visits for 2 percent of its accredited suppliers and also require all accredited suppliers to demonstrate ongoing compliance with TJC standards on an annual basis by having TJC conduct an on-site assessment or by means of electronic submission of an annual self-assessment. In contrast, federal regulations governing mammography accreditation specify the minimum number or percentage of on-site visits that should be conducted annually of accredited facilities to monitor ongoing compliance with standards and outline the activities that should be conducted during these visits.[35]

In addition, CMS guidance is not sufficient to ensure that accrediting organizations consistently identify and report serious care problems that pose immediate jeopardy to Medicare beneficiaries or suppliers' staff. CMS developed a definition of immediate jeopardy, but did not provide specific examples of the types of problems that pose an immediate health risk for ADI services. We found a difference of opinion among the accrediting organizations about the sufficiency of CMS's guidance. Representatives from TJC stated that CMS's guidance was clear, while ACR and IAC stated that the definition was too broad and stated that additional guidance is needed on the types of activities that constitute immediate jeopardy to either Medicare beneficiaries or suppliers' staff. We also found a difference of opinion about the types of activities that could constitute immediate jeopardy. For example, ACR reported that identifying metallic objects in the MRI suite would definitely constitute immediate jeopardy, whereas TJC told us that this could constitute immediate jeopardy if it was related to other pervasive lapses in safety.[36]

---

[34]IAC representatives reported that they prefer not to publish the percent of unannounced site visits as the percentages are routinely evaluated internally and may fluctuate.

[35]FDA requires each accrediting body to annually visit at least 5 percent of the facilities it accredits. However, a minimum of 5 facilities shall be visited, and visits to no more than 50 facilities are required unless identified problems indicate a need to visit more than 50 facilities. FDA requires accrediting bodies to conduct onsite visits according to a visit plan that includes assessment of quality-assurance activities, review of mammography reporting procedures, review of medical audit systems, verification of consumer complaint mechanisms, selection of a sample of clinical images for clinical image review, equipment verification, and verification that personnel specified by the facility are the ones actually performing designated personnel functions. 21 C.F.R. § 900.4(f) (2012).

[36]TJC representatives told us that while identifying metallic objects in the MRI suite may or may not constitute an immediate-jeopardy deficiency that is reported to CMS, this is always considered a serious problem that, if identified, must be corrected immediately.

ACR representatives stated that without more specific guidance, CMS relies on accrediting organizations to determine what constitutes immediate jeopardy, and noted that FDA's guidance on this topic for mammography accreditation is more helpful. Although federal regulations require the accrediting organizations to report immediate-jeopardy deficiencies of accredited suppliers to CMS within 2 business days, CMS officials reported that none had been reported since the accreditation requirement went into effect. It is unclear whether CMS's lack of guidance has contributed to the fact that no immediate-jeopardy deficiencies have been reported. For example, representatives from one accrediting organization reported that there were circumstances in which they may not report potential immediate jeopardy deficiencies to CMS because they were not certain of exactly what constituted immediate jeopardy.

Conclusions

The MIPPA accreditation requirement is an important step in helping to ensure the safety and quality of imaging services. To meet the January 1, 2012, implementation date for MIPPA's accreditation requirement, CMS focused its initial efforts on selecting accrediting organizations and ensuring that only accredited suppliers were paid. However, there are significant differences among the accrediting organizations, which arise from CMS's lack of minimum national standards. As a result, important aspects of imaging, such as qualifications of technologists and medical directors and the quality of clinical images, are difficult for CMS to monitor and assess. CMS lacks an oversight framework for evaluating the performance of selected accrediting organizations, and lacks specific guidance to help ensure that a sufficient number or percentage of mid-cycle audits occurs and that the types of serious care problems that could constitute immediate jeopardy are clear to all accrediting organizations.

Recommendations for Executive Action

To help ensure that ADI suppliers provide consistent, safe, and high-quality imaging to Medicare beneficiaries, we recommend that the Administrator of CMS take the following three actions:

- determine the content of and publish minimum national standards for the accreditation of ADI suppliers, which could include specific qualifications for supplier personnel and requiring accrediting organization review of clinical images;

- develop an oversight framework for evaluating accrediting organization performance, which could include collecting and

- analyzing information on accreditation results and conducting validation audits; and

- develop more specific requirements for accrediting organization mid-cycle audit procedures and clarify guidance on immediate-jeopardy deficiencies to ensure consistent identification and timely correction of serious care problems for the duration of accreditation.

Agency and Third Party Comments and Our Evaluation

We provided a draft of this report to HHS and to the three CMS-approved accrediting organizations for comment. In its written response, reproduced in appendix I, HHS concurred with all of our recommendations and identified actions that the department and CMS officials plan to take to implement them. Specifically, HHS stated these actions would include

- facilitating discussions with stakeholders and national experts to gather feedback on national standards for accreditation of ADI suppliers;

- developing an oversight framework for evaluating accrediting organization performance; and

- developing more specific requirements for accrediting organizations' review procedures and providing guidance and education on immediate-jeopardy deficiencies.

The three accrediting organizations also reviewed and provided comments on a draft of this report. ACR and IAC concurred with the report's findings and recommendations. IAC representatives also said that minimum standards for ADI accreditation should include a review of suppliers' interpretive reports of patient images, in addition to the other standards identified in the report. In contrast, TJC disagreed with the report's findings and methodology. A summary of TJC's specific comments and our response follows. The three accrediting organizations also provided technical comments, which we incorporated as appropriate.

TJC stated that the report's methodology was flawed and that it provided an incomplete portrayal of the necessary components of an ADI accreditation program. TJC indicated that the 11 organizations from which we obtained information on standards focused only on imaging and did not include organizations that focus more broadly on quality and safety. As a result, TJC stated that the report excluded other factors that affect quality oversight and improvement, and indicated that we lacked data to analyze the effectiveness of the different approaches used by each of the three organizations. Our purpose was not to compare the effectiveness of the three ADI accreditation programs, but rather to assess the ADI standards currently in use and determine whether CMS has adequate assurance that all accredited suppliers meet a minimum level of quality and safety. Further, we did not intend to conduct a comprehensive evaluation of TJC's overall accreditation program, which considers aspects of quality and safety that go beyond criteria outlined in MIPPA for imaging accreditation, such as examining whether a supplier creates and maintains a culture of safety and quality throughout the organization. Rather, because our study is focused on imaging in particular, we determined whether the three CMS-selected accrediting organizations use standards specific to imaging that were recommended by organizations with expertise in this area.

TJC also questioned our threshold for presenting standards that were recommended by 5 of 11 of the organizations, indicating that this represented agreement from less than 50 percent of the organizations. Because the 11 organizations have expertise in different areas of imaging, not all organizations commented on all sections of the questionnaire we sent to them. For example, the American Board of Orthopaedic Surgery recommended standards related to the qualifications of medical directors, but not procedures to ensure that equipment meets performance specifications. As a result, it would not be reasonable or appropriate to expect consensus for all recommended standards, as some standards were outside of an organization's area of expertise. We indicate in the report that the standards the 11 organizations identified do not represent the full range of possible standards for the accreditation of ADI suppliers, but rather provide a framework for comparing the standards used by the accrediting organizations selected by CMS. HHS has indicated that it plans to facilitate discussions with stakeholders and national experts to gather feedback on national standards for accreditation of ADI suppliers.

Finally, TJC stated that the report places inordinate value on image accuracy and professional credentials. We discuss those aspects of imaging in the report because they were among the nine standards that were identified by at least 5 of the 11 organizations with imaging expertise. For example, 8 of the 11 organizations believe that examining clinical images is an important aspect of accreditation for ADI services, and it is unclear how problems with image quality can be detected without reviewing images. Similarly, TJC stated that we provided no data to show that phantom testing results in better image quality in practice. Phantom image testing was recommended by 5 of the 11 organizations with imaging expertise, and has been required by FDA for over a decade to test imaging conducted by mammogram facilities under MQSA. Further, phantom images provide a standardized format against which imaging performance of various suppliers can be evaluated; this is important given that factors outside of a supplier's control, such as a patient's weight or particular health conditions, can affect a supplier's ability to produce high-quality images.

While our report assessed the standards currently in use for ADI accreditation, it is ultimately CMS's responsibility to determine the content of minimum national standards for ADI accreditation. This could include, for example, determining whether clinical image review and phantom testing should be required for ADI accreditation, a decision that could be informed by its planned discussions with stakeholders and national experts. We stand by our report and findings, and believe that by adopting our recommendations for minimum national standards, as HHS has stated it intends to do, CMS will significantly enhance its ability to ensure both imaging quality and patient safety.

We are sending copies of this report to the Secretary of Health and Human Services and relevant congressional committees. The report will also be available at no charge on the GAO website at http://www.gao.gov.

If you or your staff has any questions about this report, please contact me at (202) 512-7114 or cosgrovej@gao.gov. Contact points for our Offices of Congressional Relations and Public Affairs may be found on the last page of this report. GAO staff who made major contributions to this report are listed in appendix II.

James Cosgrove
Director, Health Care

List of Committees

The Honorable Max Baucus
Chairman
The Honorable Orrin G. Hatch
Ranking Member
Committee on Finance
United States Senate

The Honorable Fred Upton
Chairman
The Honorable Henry A. Waxman
Ranking Member
Committee on Energy and Commerce
House of Representatives

The Honorable Dave Camp
Chairman
The Honorable Sander M. Levin
Ranking Member
Committee on Ways and Means
House of Representatives

Appendix I: Comments for the Department of Health and Human Services

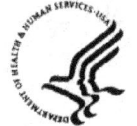

DEPARTMENT OF HEALTH & HUMAN SERVICES OFFICE OF THE SECRETARY

Assistant Secretary for Legislation
Washington, DC 20201

APR 01 2013

James C. Cosgrove
Director, Health Care
U.S. Government Accountability Office
441 G Street NW
Washington, DC 20548

Dear Mr. Cosgrove:

Attached are comments on the U.S. Government Accountability Office's (GAO) report entitled, "MEDICARE IMAGING ACCREDITATION: Establishing Minimum National Standards and an Oversight Framework Would Help Ensure Quality and Safety of Advanced Diagnostic Imaging Services" (GAO-13-246).

The Department appreciates the opportunity to review this report prior to publication.

Sincerely,

Jim R. Esquea
Assistant Secretary for Legislation

Attachment

Appendix I: Comments for the Department of Health and Human Services

GENERAL COMMENTS OF THE DEPARTMENT OF HEALTH AND HUMAN SERVICES (HHS) ON THE GOVERNMENT ACCOUNTABILITY OFFICE'S (GAO) DRAFT REPORT ENTITLED, "MEDICARE IMAGING ACCREDITATION: ESTABLISHING MINIMUM NATIONAL STANDARDS AND AN OVERSIGHT FRAMEWORK WOULD HELP ENSURE QUALITY AND SAFETY OF ADVANCED DIAGNOSTIC IMAGING SERVICES" (GAO-13-246)

GAO Recommendation
GAO recommends that CMS determine the content of and publish minimum national standards for the accreditation of ADI suppliers, which could include specific qualifications for supplier personnel and requiring accrediting organization review of clinical images.

HHS Response
HHS concurs with the recommendation to strengthen the ADI program. CMS is working to transition the ADI program from the Center for Program Integrity to the Center for Clinical Standards and Quality (CCSQ) at CMS. Moving the ADI program to CCSQ will more closely align it with ongoing standards and enforcement activities. Once the transition occurs on April 1, 2013, CMS intends to facilitate discussion with stakeholders and national experts to gather feedback on national standards for the accreditation of ADI suppliers.

GAO Recommendation
GAO recommends that CMS develop an oversight framework for evaluation accrediting organization performance, which could include collecting and analyzing information on accreditation results and conducting validation audits.

HHS Response
HHS concurs with this recommendation. We will work within statutory and regulatory authority to develop an oversight framework for evaluating accrediting organization performance and will consider collecting and analyzing information on accreditation results and conducting validation audits. To further strengthen our oversight, we plan to revise and expand our regulations at 42 CFR 488 to provide stronger oversight of accrediting organizations to include accrediting organizations of ADI suppliers.

GAO Recommendation
GAO recommends that CMS develop more specific requirements for accrediting organization mid-cycle audit procedures and clarify guidance on immediate jeopardy deficiencies to ensure consistent identification and timely correction of serious problems for the duration of accreditation.

HHS Response
HHS concurs with this recommendation. As part of our overall effort to develop an oversight framework for evaluating accrediting organization performance in this area, we will evaluate our current requirements and develop more specific requirements for accrediting organization review procedures. In addition, we will provide guidance and education on immediate jeopardy deficiencies to ensure consistent identification and timely correction of serious care problems for the duration of the accreditation period. Our experience with oversight of other accrediting organizations under 42 CFR 488 in our regulations will serve us well in our work in this area as well.

Appendix II: GAO Contact and Staff Acknowledgments

GAO Contact	James Cosgrove, (202) 512-7114 or cosgrovej@gao.gov
Staff Acknowledgments	In addition to the contact named above, Phyllis Thorburn, Assistant Director; William Black; Kye Briesath; William A. Crafton; Beth Morrison; Jennifer Whitworth; and Rachael Wojnowicz made key contributions to this report.

GAO's Mission	The Government Accountability Office, the audit, evaluation, and investigative arm of Congress, exists to support Congress in meeting its constitutional responsibilities and to help improve the performance and accountability of the federal government for the American people. GAO examines the use of public funds; evaluates federal programs and policies; and provides analyses, recommendations, and other assistance to help Congress make informed oversight, policy, and funding decisions. GAO's commitment to good government is reflected in its core values of accountability, integrity, and reliability.
Obtaining Copies of GAO Reports and Testimony	The fastest and easiest way to obtain copies of GAO documents at no cost is through GAO's website (http://www.gao.gov). Each weekday afternoon, GAO posts on its website newly released reports, testimony, and correspondence. To have GAO e-mail you a list of newly posted products, go to http://www.gao.gov and select "E-mail Updates."
Order by Phone	The price of each GAO publication reflects GAO's actual cost of production and distribution and depends on the number of pages in the publication and whether the publication is printed in color or black and white. Pricing and ordering information is posted on GAO's website, http://www.gao.gov/ordering.htm. Place orders by calling (202) 512-6000, toll free (866) 801-7077, or TDD (202) 512-2537. Orders may be paid for using American Express, Discover Card, MasterCard, Visa, check, or money order. Call for additional information.
Connect with GAO	Connect with GAO on Facebook, Flickr, Twitter, and YouTube. Subscribe to our RSS Feeds or E-mail Updates. Listen to our Podcasts. Visit GAO on the web at www.gao.gov.
To Report Fraud, Waste, and Abuse in Federal Programs	Contact: Website: http://www.gao.gov/fraudnet/fraudnet.htm E-mail: fraudnet@gao.gov Automated answering system: (800) 424-5454 or (202) 512-7470
Congressional Relations	Katherine Siggerud, Managing Director, siggerudk@gao.gov, (202) 512-4400, U.S. Government Accountability Office, 441 G Street NW, Room 7125, Washington, DC 20548
Public Affairs	Chuck Young, Managing Director, youngc1@gao.gov, (202) 512-4800 U.S. Government Accountability Office, 441 G Street NW, Room 7149 Washington, DC 20548

Please Print on Recycled Paper.

www.ingramcontent.com/pod-product-compliance
Lightning Source LLC
Chambersburg PA
CBHW081812170526
45167CB00008B/3414